YOGA BEYOND THE POSES

Tantra YOGA

*The Ultimate Beginner's Guide
to Discover Tantra Yoga, Yoga Philosophy,
and Magic!*

Shreyanada Natha

Cover & design

Mattias Långström

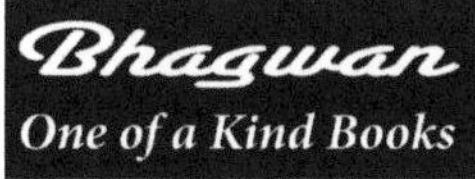

YOGA BEYOND THE POSES

Tantra

YOGA

*The Ultimate Beginner's Guide
to Discover Tantra Yoga, Yoga Philosophy,
and Magic!*

Shreyanada Natha

ISBN 9789198839258

✸✸✸

Copyright © Mattias Långström

2024

2 FREE PREMIUM BONUS!

#1. *Download the* **AUDIOBOOK** *at the back of the book!*

#2. *Download* **CHAKRA-INDEX IN COLOR** *here!*

SCAN QR-CODE or go to:

https://bit.ly/47wdFVZ

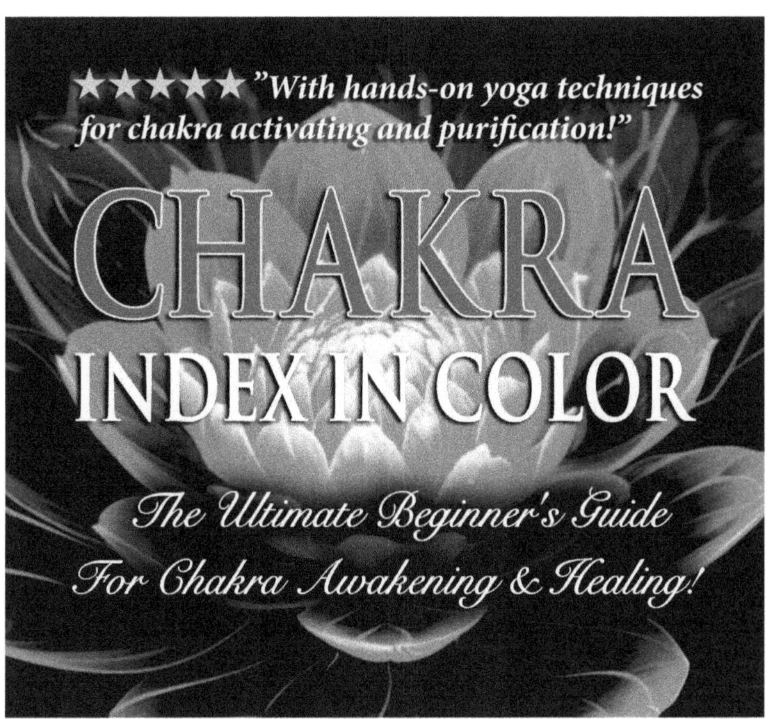

FREE PREMIUM Audiobook
Authentic Yoga Nidra Meditation – Anahata Chakra Awakening!

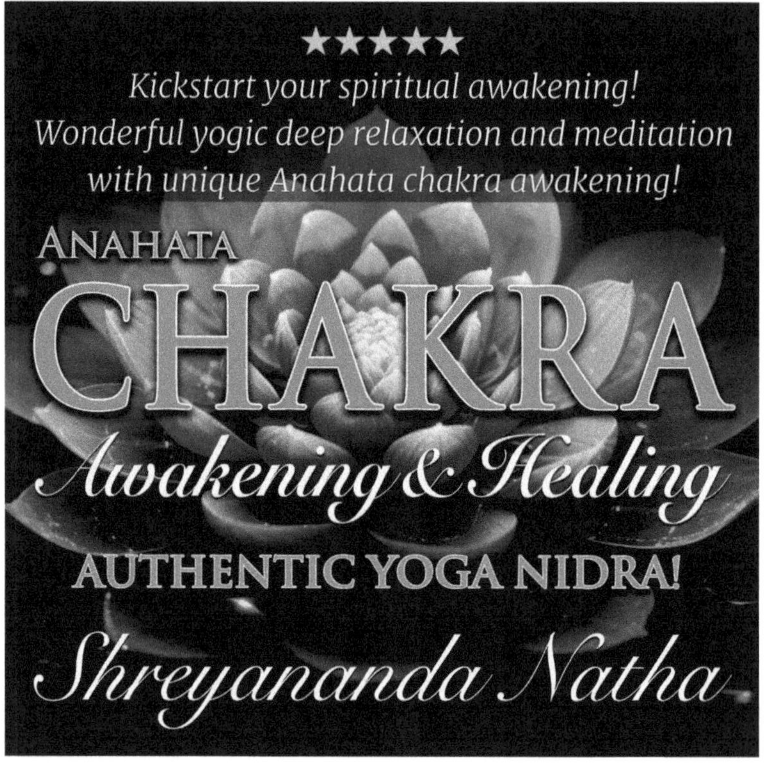

*Download the **AUDIOBOOK** at the back of the book!*

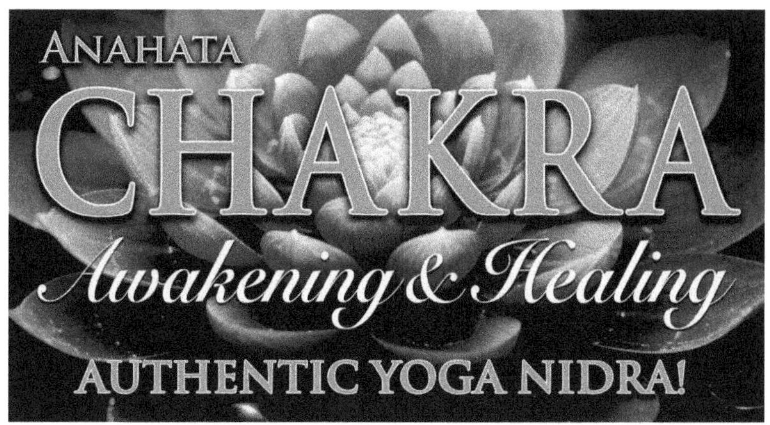

Kickstart your spiritual awakening! Wonderful yogic deep relaxation and meditation with unique Anahata chakra awakening and healing.

PRESENTATION

Yoga Nidra, or yogic sleep, is a unique meditation process that`s powerfully profound and healing for body, mind, and spirit.

Practitioners are led into a state of deep relaxation and the experience of our chakra system.

Yoga Nidra offers extensive benefits, yet it is one of the most straightforward yoga practices.

All you have to do is put on your most comfortable clothes, find a quiet space, lie down on your back, and play the meditation.

Yoga Beyond the Poses – Tantra Yoga
The Ultimate Beginner's Guide to Discover Tantra Yoga, Yoga Philosophy, and Magic!
Including A Premium Audiobook: Yoga Nidra Meditation – Anahata Chakra Awakening And Healing!

The book describes Tantra yoga – Yoga Philosophy and Magic. Its origin and mystery are from the ground up. It penetrates deeply but remains easy to read, educational, and understandable. A must on the bookshelf for anyone interested in Tantra yoga – Yoga Philosophy and Magic who quickly wants to know more.

The book is part of a series of seven yoga books, Yoga Beyond the Poses: The Ultimate Beginner's Guide to Yoga, that delve into the seven key areas of yoga.

INCLUDING A PREMIUM AUDIOBOOK: AUTHENTIC YOGA NIDRA MEDITATION – ANAHATA CHAKRA AWAKENING & HEALING!
Kickstart your spiritual awakening! Wonderful yogic deep relaxation and meditation with unique Anahata chakra awakening and healing.

Yoga Nidra, or yogic sleep, is a unique meditation process that's powerfully profound and healing for body, mind, and spirit. Practitioners are led into a state of deep relaxation

and the experience of our chakra system. Yoga Nidra offers extensive benefits, yet it is one of the most straightforward yoga practices. All you have to do is put on your most comfortable clothes, find a quiet space, lie down on your back, and play the meditation. –
Download the audiobook at the back of the book!

ABOUT THE BOOK SERIES
YOGA BEYOND THE POSES: *The Ultimate Beginner's Guide to Yoga!*

The book is part of a seven-book yoga series, Yoga Beyond the Poses: The Ultimate Beginner's Guide to Yoga, that delve into yoga's seven most important areas. They are straightforward to read, educational, and fascinating. A must on the bookshelf for anyone interested in yoga who quickly wants to know more.

MY NAME AND MY MISSION
Shreyananda Natha was the name I was given when I was initiated into the Natha Order and received the master mantra – the Shodasi mantra, after studying yoga and tantra for over twelve years, the highest mantra in yoga and tantra. It means "he who knows".

After practicing yoga and meditation continuously for over twenty years, having a yoga school for many years, and leading studies for yoga teachers, I wanted to get out more wi-

*dely with yoga into our whole society, out of the small yoga
room. Spread the knowledge of yoga, our chakra system, and
Kundalini Shakti to anyone who will listen. What needed
to be added were educational fact books on yoga that didn't
just skim the surface or deal with the author's private life. So
it became my Sankalpa, my magical wish, and my mission
to create exciting yoga books that everyone should be able to
read and enjoy. To show how we can apply and use yoga in
different areas of life and achieve success and health. Here
and now.*

*If you like my books, feel free to follow me on my social
media, share and like, tell your friends about the books, and
write an honest review; one or two lines don't matter. All
support is precious.*

Thanks!

THE AUTHOR

Shreyananda Natha is the author of popular and best-selling yoga books. He has, among other things, written one of the most comprehensive books about yoga – EVERYTHING ABOUT YOGA and the study book – TEACHING YOGA AND MEDITATION BEYOND THE POSES. He is also a certified yoga and meditation teacher according to the EYTF international guidelines. He has undergone multi-year yoga teacher training under the guidance of Swami Omananda at Satyananda Ashram and holds the highest initiation in the tantric Natha order. He frequently travels to Asia and India to learn and gain knowledge and inspiration. He has immersed himself in tantric rituals and is known for his extensive knowledge of yoga, deep relaxation, and meditation.

"There is no authority that can say what yoga is. When you surrender yourself completely and fully and experience yoga without limitations and doubts, the true encounter with yoga occurs when you become one with the true experience within you. Only then will you understand what yoga is – for you. When you are no longer limited by neatness, shyness, and artificial thought patterns that act as a filter between you and the transformation. Yoga is a cultural-historical wealth still passed on from teacher to student and helps man find his way back to his true nature. It opens us up and attracts awareness. It strengthens our self-esteem, and our person's entire spectrum of possibilities suddenly becomes visible.

Yoga is not difficult or strange. You don't have to become a vegan, a monk, or be able to stand on your head. You just need to do your yoga regularly; the rest will take care of itself. You can use yoga and meditation to feel better, both physically and mentally, but also to achieve success and develop in all areas of life – here and now."

Good luck!

Namasté

I want to thank the teachers and students I've had over the years who have made my journey with yoga so enjoyable. Thank you for all the inspiration you have given me and for making this book possible. The yoga masters who no longer live among us – live on with each new person who immerses themselves in the yoga tradition.

Sri Swami Sivananda, Sri Swami Satyananda, Sri Tirumalai Krishnamacharya, Sri Swami Vishnudevananda, Sri K. Pattabhi Jois, Osho, Swami Nirdosha, Swami Omananda, Swami Janakananda, Ole Schmidt, Turiya, Maryam Abrishami and Sanna Kuittinen.

People who all searched for answers to what they sensed through an activated Ajna chakra. In yoga, they have learned the principles behind the universe, the collective consciousness, and the creative force, Kundalini Shakti. The duality behind everything, both what we see and what we don't see. Together, we are helped to pass on the previously secret knowledge about our gunas, nadis, and chakras to all who want to become a Rishi.

Aum Shri Durgayai Namaha

Shreyananda Natha

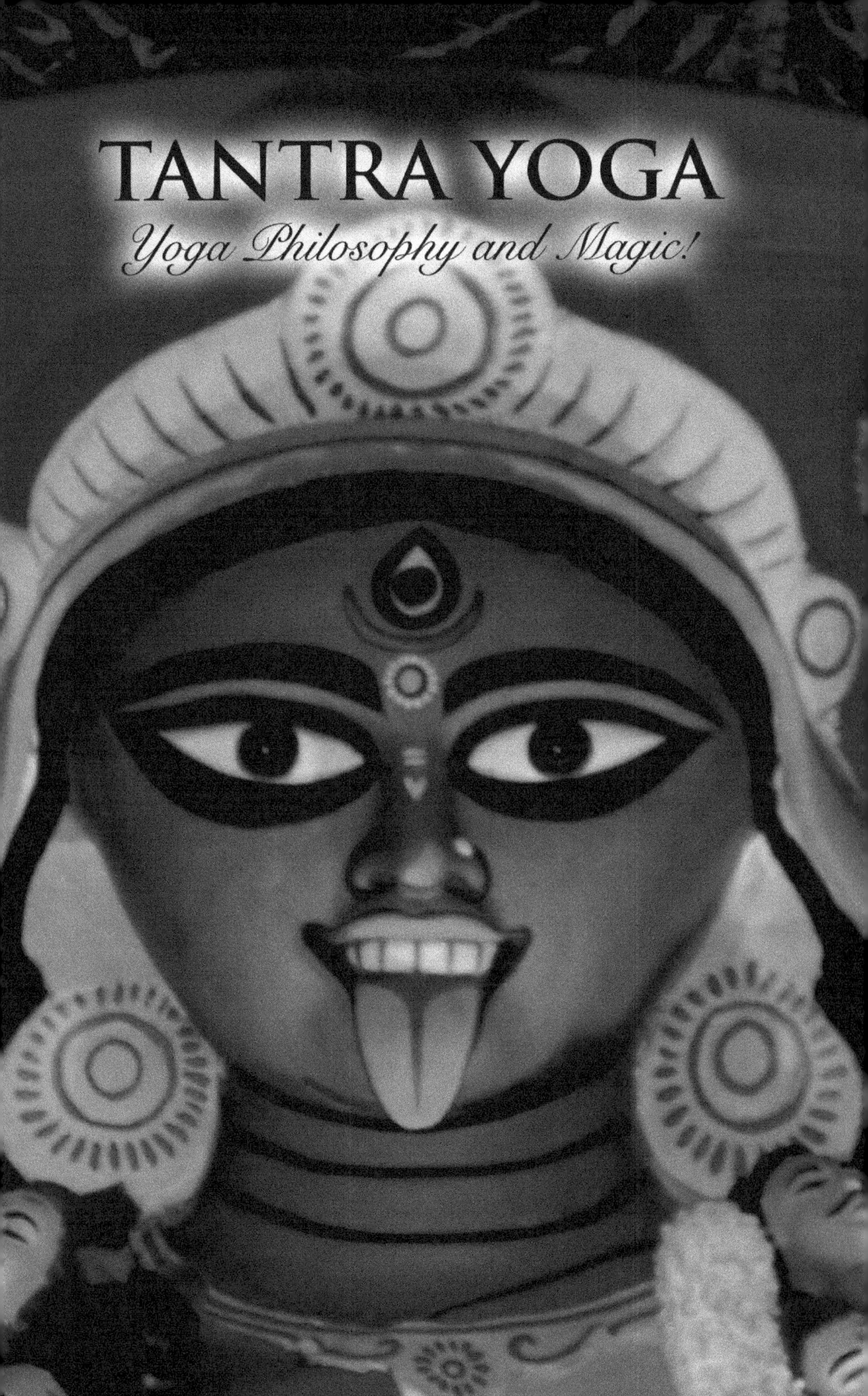
TANTRA YOGA
Yoga Philosophy and Magic!

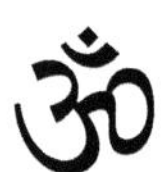

TANTRA YOGA

TANTRA, MANTRA & YANTRA

The word tantra refers to those religious, literary works in which mysticism and magic play the leading role and form the ritual books belonging to the mysticism of later Hinduism.

Tantra books are intended to guide the use of magical and mysterious formulas and are often in the form of dialogues between Shiva and Durga. The word tantra comes from Sanskrit and combines the words tanoti and trayati, which can be translated as expansion and liberation. Tantra is about expanding the mind and releasing the dormant potential energy in man. Tantra sadhana – different tantric rituals – all evoke Kundalini Shakti differently.

To expand the mind, we must learn not to be controlled by our sensory experiences. When our senses and ego govern us, we categorize all our experiences into what we "like" and" do not like," which are called raga and does. This categorization leads to suffering and inhibits our development and ability to see pure, actual knowledge. As we develop and expand the mind, we gradually build our intuitive ability, which is the source of accurate, eternal, and correct knowledge.

Daily, we perceive and take in our surroundings through our senses. If we instead learn to see, feel, listen, and turn the mind inwards, we can create an inner experience about ourselves and thus expand the mind. By releasing the energy (Shakti) and merging it with consciousness (Shiva), we create a homogeneous consciousness and experience Kundalini, which is the very purpose of tantra. The difference between tantra and most other spiritual and philosophical paths is that in tantra, you do not set up many rules that you have to live by.

Everyone has an opportunity to develop, regardless of where they are. One can be sensualist or spiritualist, atheist or theist, poor or rich, strong or weak; the road is for everyone to discover. There are a total of sixty-four different tantras, and each one describes a different approach to mind control and expansion. Tantric techniques are often mistaken for being dirty and bizarre when alcohol, drugs, and sex are included in specific exercises and rituals. However, it is not used as a means of pleasure but to expand the mind.

Tantra describes Shakti, the subtle form of energy, as a coiled snake at the bottom of the body at the end of the spine, at the Mooladhara chakra. Shiva, the pure consciousness, is said to have its seat on top of the head in the Sahasrara chakra. To awaken the Kundalini energy, which in most people is dormant, one must first increase the flow and amount of prana, the vital energy down to the Mooladhara chakra. Then, Kundalini Shakti can be directed up to the Sahasrara chakra. On its way up the spine, Kundalini Shakti passes six chakras or energy pools. When Kundalini Shakti rises, they are charged with energy. The chakras act as nodes for our nadis energy channels, which vibrate at different intensities. Chakras carry dormant creative forces partially evident in our daily lives and whose full potential can only emerge when Kundalini Shakti have passed through them on their way up to Shiva.

Tantric exercises are divided into three steps in the form of upasana or worship:

Shuddhi – purification of the gross, subtle and psychic elements or tattwas.
Sthiti – enlightenment by concentration achieved by purifying the elements.
Arpana – insight into the cosmic consciousness.

Tantric exercises can be easily distinguished from other non-tantric exercises by the sacred formulas, symbols, and rituals. We want to attract higher subtle forces and our inner forces through worship and traditions. Tattwa shuddhi is one of the tantric rituals.

FIRST STEP – CLEANING THE ELEMENT
One of the first introductory tantric rituals is tattwa shudd-

hi, also known as bhuta shuddhi, which aims to purify our elements.

In tantra, tattwa/bhuta shuddhi transforms the pranic flow from our elements so it returns to the original unmanifested form – Shakti. As long as the prana flows in our external organs and is fixed in our elements, our consciousness will be limited to the external world. The energy / consciousness is thus improved and modified to our physical body through our elements. By releasing it, we can also make it expand.

The first step towards expansion is purifying our basic physical, mental, psychic, and pranic structures. In yoga, various purifying techniques are aimed at this: prana shuddhi, nadi shuddhi, vak shuddhi, manas shuddhi, etc. But the practice of tattwa / bhuta shuddhi, according to the ancient tantras, is comprehensive. The techniques used in tattwa shuddhi are:

Nyasa – concentration on the body.

Prana prathishta – is the placement of life and prana in the mandala.

Panchopchara – five things sacrificed in the worship of tattwan.

Japa – mantra repetition.

In many ancient tantric texts, tattwa shuddhi is described as an essential technique to move development forward and gain greater insight. Tattwa shuddhi strengthens our personal experiences of energy and pure consciousness. It is not enough to "know" intellectually that all matter originates in pure consciousness; it must be experienced. Personal experience is the core of tantra and can be made possible with the help of tattwa shuddhi.

By focusing on tattwa yantras, we increase the prana in the body and affect each chakra. Each tattwa is tied to a chakra. Charging each chakra prepares the awakening of the Kundalini Shakti and facilitates its path up to the Sahasrara chakra. Tattwa shuddhi also develops our ability to concentrate (dharana), which leads to spontaneous meditation (dhyana), which in turn leads to awareness of the subtle essence behind matter and form (tattwa jnana).

BRIEF DESCRIPTION OF TATTWA SHUDDHI

With the help of meditation and self-reflection, the elements that make up the mind and body are purified and transformed. Tattwa shuddhi is a dynamic form of meditation and self-reflection. It is not a passive form where you must focus on the same symbol for a long time. During the implementation of tattwa shuddhi, one quickly deepens the mind by creating images of tattwa yantras (geometric images of the elements), Papa Purusha (the sinful man), and the mandala of Prana Shakti (the form of the creative energy).

You start the exercise by creating a mental image of the elements and their respective yantra in the body. You witness how the elements are born from each other, and you thus sink deeper into yourself. When one discovers the universal cosmic energy within, one uses the power to heal inner imbalances. With the help of a higher state of consciousness and a stronger mind, it is easier to heal imbalances. After this, an internal image of the elements is again created, but in reverse order. Towards the end, one visualizes an image of prana shakti, the energy manifested through the elements. Finally, apply bhasma or ash to the body.

Tattwa shuddhi can be used to enter a meditative state or as a complete sadhana.

It would help if you had practiced Hatha yoga and ajapa japa for a long time to get the most out of the exercise. The mind and body must be in good condition. You must be able to sit still for a long time without the mind being disturbed by the surroundings. Just before the exercise, it is a crucial preparation to turn the mind inward, which is best done with the help of pranayamas and trataka. You should also have a good knowledge of the location of the chakras in the body and how the prana moves along the sushumna. If you are ill, you should wait until you have recovered before practicing tattwa shuddhi.

CLEANING PROCESS

Tattwa shuddhi is a process that cleanses the elements of our body and purifies the senses connected to those elements. The sense of hearing is purified using mantra repetition; the sight by observing yantras and mandalas; the feeling and our tactile nerves by applying bhasma or ash to the body; the sense of smell by breathing exercises; and the sense of taste by eating sattvic food or by fasting.

Tattwa shuddhi cleanses not only our physical body but also the layers of our bodies. In addition to our physical body, we have several other bodies relating to the invisible parts of the mind that are affected by samskaras (latent impressions), which create sankalpa and vikalpa (thoughts / counter-thoughts) in our conscious mind.

Imbalances in the various bodies manifest themselves in the form of anxiety, distress, depression, and fear. We often find it difficult to cure these conditions in the same way as physical illnesses. In the long run, these imbalances affect our life and our personality. Our body is an extension of our mind, and each affects the other. Since the mind controls our body and its functions, it is as essential to purify your mental mind as your physical body.

In tantra, it is said that no action or thought is unclean or wrong—the unclean lies in false perception and judgment.

Through the sadhana, we can come to an understanding of this and thus fight it. Without purifying the subtle levels of the mind, reaching higher levels of consciousness is impossible. An unclean mind cannot focus or concentrate. By harmonizing the flow of prana in the body, separating the intellect and ego from the consciousness, one can purify the different levels of the mind so that one becomes the experiencer and the witness simultaneously.

CLEANING OF THE ELEMENT

Tattwa shuddhi is a unique technique because it purifies the whole person from the coarsest layers to the most subtle. The first step in the cleansing process is to wash and cleanse the physical body, apply bhasma or ash, and fast and control food intake. Tantra emphasizes the importance of doing all everyday chores with awareness and presence. Everything you do, how you sit, walk, talk, wash, etc., reflects your state of mind. Tattwa shuddhi is thus a purification process that covers all twenty-four hours of the day. However, the first step in physical purity is more about discipline than raising awareness.

The second step in the process purifies the subtle levels. You use your mind and prana. Internal forces are aroused and controlled by the elements. By refining the elements, the energy increases so that they can vibrate harmoniously, which creates a balance that leads to an increased inner awareness.

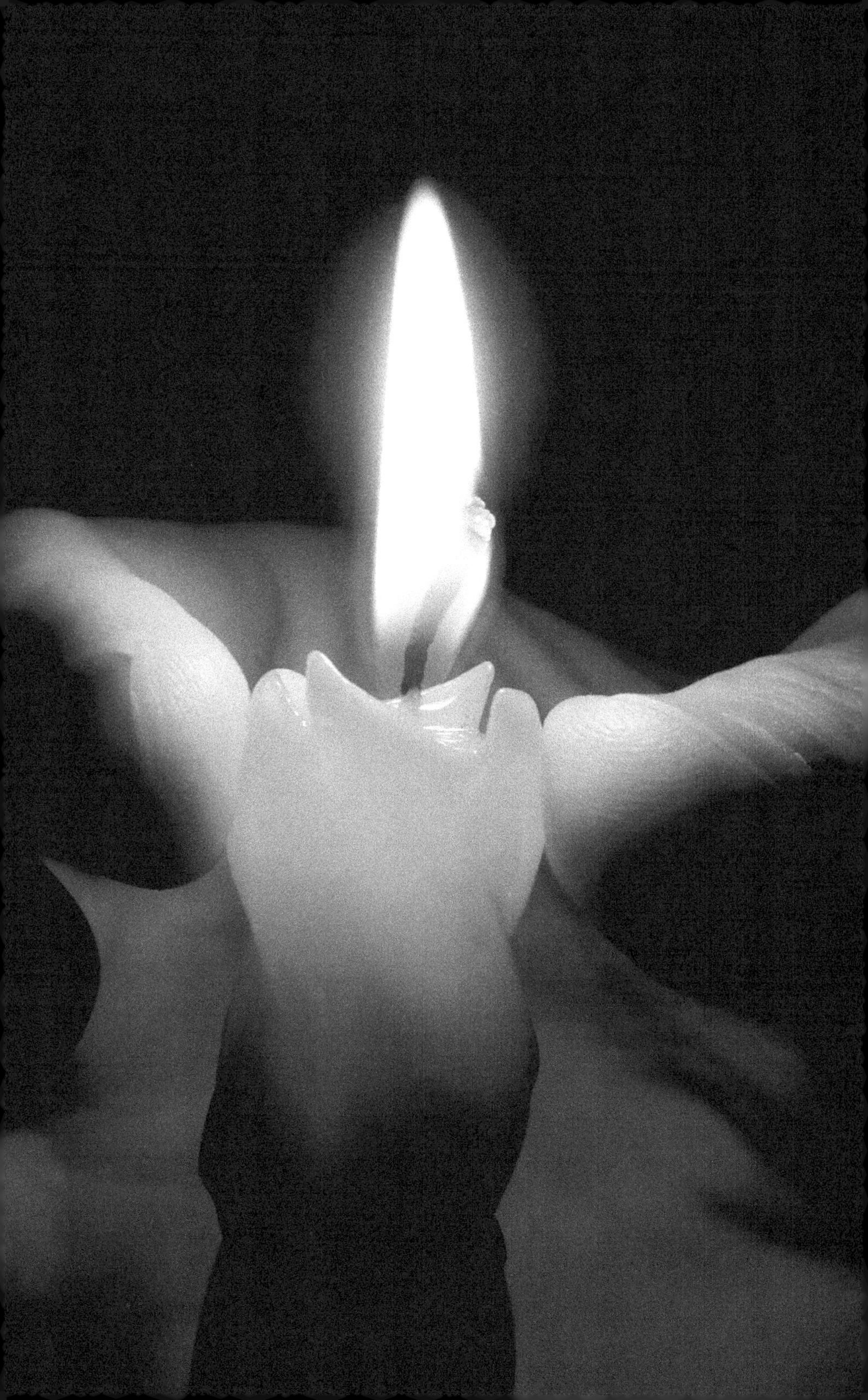

By repeating the bija mantra and visualizing the yantra of each tattwa, one can dissolve deeply rooted samskaras and archetypes that prevent us from experiencing infinite consciousness.

PRANA SHAKTI

In our body, the prana moves in a specific pattern, meaning vibrations are created at different frequency levels. The vibrational frequencies build up our physical body and our subtle organs. We can see and feel the bodily organs and their constituents while the delicate organs are experienced. In tantra and yoga, these delicate organs are chakras, nadis, Kundalini Shakti, chitta Shakti, prana vayu and pancha tattwa.

The prana exists in the microcosm and macrocosm. Without it, we would not function or exist. We would not have the ability to see, hear, or move. Most of us have too little flow of prana in our body, which leads to fatigue and exhaustion. The cosmic prana in our body is represented by Kundalini Shakti, which has its seat in the Mooladhara chakra. When its full potential is awakened, it rises along the central nervous system of our physical body, which in our pranic body is called the sushumna nadi. Kundalini Shakti also manifests itself in our more significant six chakras.

Each chakra consists of one element. In Mooladhara there are elements of the earth – prithvi tattwa; in Swadhisthana elements of water – apas tattwa; in Manipura elements of fire – agni tattwa; in Anahata elements of air – vayu tattwa; and in Vishuddhi elements of ether or space – akasha tattwa. The element that controls the chakra reveals the frequency at which the chakra vibrates. Our entire consciousness, thoughts, and actions are governed by the degree of activity of the chakra. Pingala nadi supplies chakras with energy, and Kundalini Shakti activates them to their full potential. When our chakras are only partially activated, we become limited in acting and experiencing. In tattwa shuddhi, we affect each chakra directly by concentrating on each tattwa.

MANDALA BY PRANA SHAKTI

In tantra, there is a tradition of symbolizing the various aspects of man in the form of mandalas. Mandalas represent the human subconscious and unconscious mind. Concentrating on these images can relax samskaras or archetypes that stand in the way of our creativity and knowledge. In tattwa shuddhi sadhana, a picture of prana Shakti is created as a beautiful goddess who has a powerful effect on us.

Prana Shakti, as a goddess, is red. Red is a base color that stands for raja guna. The color also symbolizes the dynamic quality of prana. Her six arms represent the efficiency she has in everything she undertakes. She holds a tool in each hand that illustrates different aspects of human existence. Her three eyes stand for prophecy, and the lotus flower she sits on for developing powers and siddhis.

ANTAH KARANA

Antah karana is man's inner tool and consists of four parts: buddhi (intellect), ahamkara (ego), manas (thoughts and counter-thoughts), and chitta (memory). According to tantra and yoga, these four are the core of consciousness, which acts from the outside. Antah karana is unique and can only be found in humans. In lower life forms (animals and plant species), antah karana exists only as a precursor. Plants and animals act instinctively, not based on ego, intellect, or thoughts. Antah karana is what sets man apart from other species.

Through antah karana, the human consciousness interprets, classifies and perceives everything that concerns the past, present and future. It is a recipient who receives and sends out impressions. In antah karana, in addition to the knowledge of this life and what happens here, there is also the knowledge of the universe and cosmos. This knowledge is often unmanifested and dormant in humans. Refining the frequency of antah karana is part of human evolution.

Antah karana is an instrument built up through all our incarnations. It carries all the impressions of our past lives. Antah karana determines the individual's future actions based on previous experiences and knowledge. These experiences and expertise are often unconscious unless we develop our inner vision and experience of the cosmos. Through tantric techniques, we can learn to see and control antah karana, which is part of our evolution.

DIMENSIONS OF THE MIND

In yoga, the mind is divided into four parts: jagriti (conscious mind), swapana (unconscious mind), sushpati (subconscious mind) and turya (our transcendental mind). In modern psychology, only the first three are mentioned.

Antah karana acts based on the conscious, subconscious, and unconscious mind. Manas and chitta, which are part of the conscious and subconscious mind, control thoughts and actions on the conscious and subconscious plane. Buddhi and ahamkara constantly exist to varying degrees in the conscious, subconscious, and unconscious mind. Since all of these have arisen from the same principle, Shakti, they influence each other intensively.

The three gunas, sattva, rajas, and tamas, lay the foundation for antah karana. These three cosmic principles significantly influence manas, chitta, and buddhi and thus affect our experiences. The fourth sense, turya, is unaffected by the interplay between the three gunas. Turya can only be developed by refining antah karana through sadhana. In tattwa shuddhi, we learn to perceive antah karana and use its full potential for further spiritual development.

BUDDHI

Buddhi is the principle that most closely resembles pure consciousness. It motivates us to follow our dharma. Sattvic buddhi is characterized by wisdom, happiness, perseverance, calm, self-control and discernment. Under the influence of rajas, some defects occur, which means that the ability to distinguish deteriorates, and even actions are affected by wrong knowledge and avidya. A tamasic buddhi acts under the ego, which is judgmental and permeated by misinterpretations of the outside world. In tattwa shuddhi, the principle of buddhi is meditated on sattvic. It removes the qualities of rajas and tamas that stand in the way of sattvic buddhi.

AHAMKARA

Aham means "I," and ahamkara is the ego or what one experiences as the "self." The ego is the core of individualism, which makes us identify with matter. Ahamkara is very subtle. At the same time as the ego binds man to objective experiences, it is the core that must be opened to experience unity. Without the ego, man would not be aware of his existence. On the conscious plane, the ego acts through our physical body, senses, and mind. On the subconscious plane, it works through our astral body and dreams. During deep sleep, the ego withdraws, while during meditation, it functions as the inner consciousness.

Sattvic ahamkara acts as a catalyst for self-realization.

Ahamkara usually takes up the comrades and underlying experiences from the subconscious mind, but in a sattvic state, this stops. Rajasic ahamkara raises the identification with the "self," leading to restlessness and a constant need to do something. A tamasic ahamkara strengthens painful and negative samskaras, which causes fear and doubt. Through tattwa shuddhi, we can see how the ego works and thus stop identifying with it.

MANAS AND CHITTA

Manas and chitta represent the external mind: thoughts in our waking state and during dreams. Chitta is the core of all experiences in the form of samskaras, archetypes, and memories. Manas, i.e., our thoughts, are chitta's tools that co-exist and by which archetypes and memories are expressed. Manas and chitta do not work individually but are influenced by both buddhi and ahamkara. Our manas are steady, focused, and concentrated in a sattvic state. Our senses are activated under the influence of rajas, creating an imbalance in our intellect. Tamasic manas make the intellect and the senses sluggish and inactive.

When chitta is in a sattvic state, our senses are withdrawn so that consciousness remains undisturbed. Under the influence of rajas, rajasic awakened samskaras in chitta in the form of vikalpa (fantasy) and viparayaya (wrong knowledge). In that state, chitta contains cohabitation, knowledge and ignorance, passion and freedom. When tamas prevail in chitta, unwanted samskaras will emerge as vasanas (deep-rooted desires).

The coexistence of a negative nature can only be eliminated through reflection, dharana, and dhyana. Tattwa shuddhi helps us enter meditation, which aims to liberate the consciousness. Only then can we reflect on the structure of the elements and influence them.

PANCHA TATTWA – THE FIVE ELEMENTS

All matter comprises five elements, akasha, vayu, agni, apas and prithvi. The elements lay the foundation for the creation and make it last. The elements affect every aspect of our lives, thoughts, and actions. In yoga, it is essential to learn how these elements work to be able to control and influence them and our lives. In tantric texts, the science behind the elements is described.

The elements form a chain where they are born from each other. Akasha is the first element of the process. Akasha consists of subtle matter and energy, which rests in consciousness. When the energy in akasha begins to vibrate, movement is created, and vayu tattwa takes shape. Vayu stands for the movement that permeates everything. The intense movement creates heat, which causes the next element in the joint (agni) to be made. Agni tattwa has a slower vibration than vayu. It allows the heat to cool down and form apas and water elements. The vibration and movement of the apas are minimal. The last element, prithvi, occurs when the movement/vibration is further reduced. Apas solidify and become the elements of the earth. The elements should extend pure consciousness, not separate existing parts.

During evolution, tattwas have been further developed through tanmatras. Tanmatra is the quality through which tattwas are perceived. Akasha is perceived through shaba tanmatra (sound), vayu through sparsha tanmatra (feeling), agni through roopa tanmatra (vision), apas through rasa tanmatra (taste) and prithvi through gandha tanmatra (smell). We are created from the roughest form of the elements when we are born. In tattwa shuddhi, we have an experience of the elements in their subtle form to develop spiritually.

The Patanjali Yoga Sutras state that each element consists of five different characters. To take control of the elements, one must practice samyama, a combination of concentration, meditation, and samadhi. Patanjali called this bhuta jaya "knowledge of the elements." The first character of the five elements is the rough form related to experiences we take through our senses: sound, touch, form, taste, and smell. The second character relates to the quality of the elements:

- *The liquid property of water.*
- *The heat of the fire.*
- *The movement of air.*
- *The space of ether.*

The third character is the subtle form of tanmatras. Here, tattwas are experienced in quiet sounds, sensations, form, smell and taste and are often called mental visions. The fourth aspect of the elements relates to the three gunas (sattva, rajas, and tamas), which are an essential part of the elements. One should strive to transform the qualities of rajasic and tamasic into more sattvic to develop spiritually. Tattwa shuddhi enables this change. The fifth aspect of the elements is called arthavattwa, which stands for the actual goal of the elements. The scriptures describe that it is for the liberation and enjoyment of consciousness from matter that the elements have developed.

The elements are characterized by shaba (sound) and warn (color) and are created by the vibration in the component. The color refers to the energy frequency of the element. Akasha is black, as the vibration is minimal. Vayu vibrates in the frequency of blue, agni in red, apas in white and prithvi in yellow. The second manifestation of the energy of the elements is sound in the form of bija mantras. Bija mantra for akasha is Ham, for vayu – Yam, agni – Ram, apas – Vam and prithvi – Lam.

Sound and color together build the form of energy. Akasha is experienced as a circle, vayu as a hexagon, agni as an inverted triangle, apas as a horizontal crescent moon and prithvi as a yellow square.

AKASHA TATTWA – the element of space.

Akasha can be described as the space or emptiness between two objects or matter. Akasha is the most subtle of all the elements and is almost motionless. It stands for the whole spectrum of sounds, from the rough to the quiet, and acts as a carrier for the sound. The vibration of the element is so subtle that it cannot be experienced with external senses. It is said that ether moves at a higher speed than sound. Akasha tattwa is boundless and permeates the entire cosmos; therefore, it has the shape of a circle. It is not of matter as we know it and cannot be experienced physically. Tattwa jnanis has discovered akasha by refining the rough mind. Because of this quality, tantra has described the element as mental (not physical) and the "space of the mind" behind closed eyes, called chidakasha. Tattwa akasha stands for the space in the body between our organs. On a mental level, tattwa akasha controls man's emotions and passions. The best time for meditation and concentration is when akasha flows in the body, which happens about five minutes every hour. The element has its seat on top of the head. Mentally, it relates to our unconscious mind, and its psychic centers are the Vishuddhi chakra. The spiritual experience created by the element is jnana loka and anandamaya kosha.

VAYU TATTWA – the element of air.

Vayu can be translated as air. The element is gray-blue and is symbolized by a hexagon. Vayu stands for kinetic energy in all its forms: electrical, chemical, vital, and prana. Its quality is movement, and it controls all movement qualities in the body, including prana, apana, samana, udana, and vyana. Vayu is responsible for our ability to experience physical touch. When we develop the mind for touch, we can experience the feeling of energy in us and around us. Even vayu is physically invisible. The element can be described as "energy in motion." Movement creates change, which means this element can cause stability and instability in humans and the environment. Vayu has its seat between the heart and the eyebrows. Mentally, the element relates to the subconscious mind. Its psychic center is the Anahata chakra. The spiritual experience of vayu is maha loka and vijnamaya kosha, our intuitive body.

AGNI TATTWA – the element of fire.

Agni or fire is called tejas, meaning "to sharpen." The element is primarily energy and is experienced as light. With the help of light, we can see the shape. The sense organ that agni relates to is the eye, which allows us to see. Form or matter is the core of the emergence of our ego. The ego identifies with form, which leads to attachment to things. Agni tattwa is thus not only the first manifestation of the form and the stage when ahamkara begins to grow. The element wears the

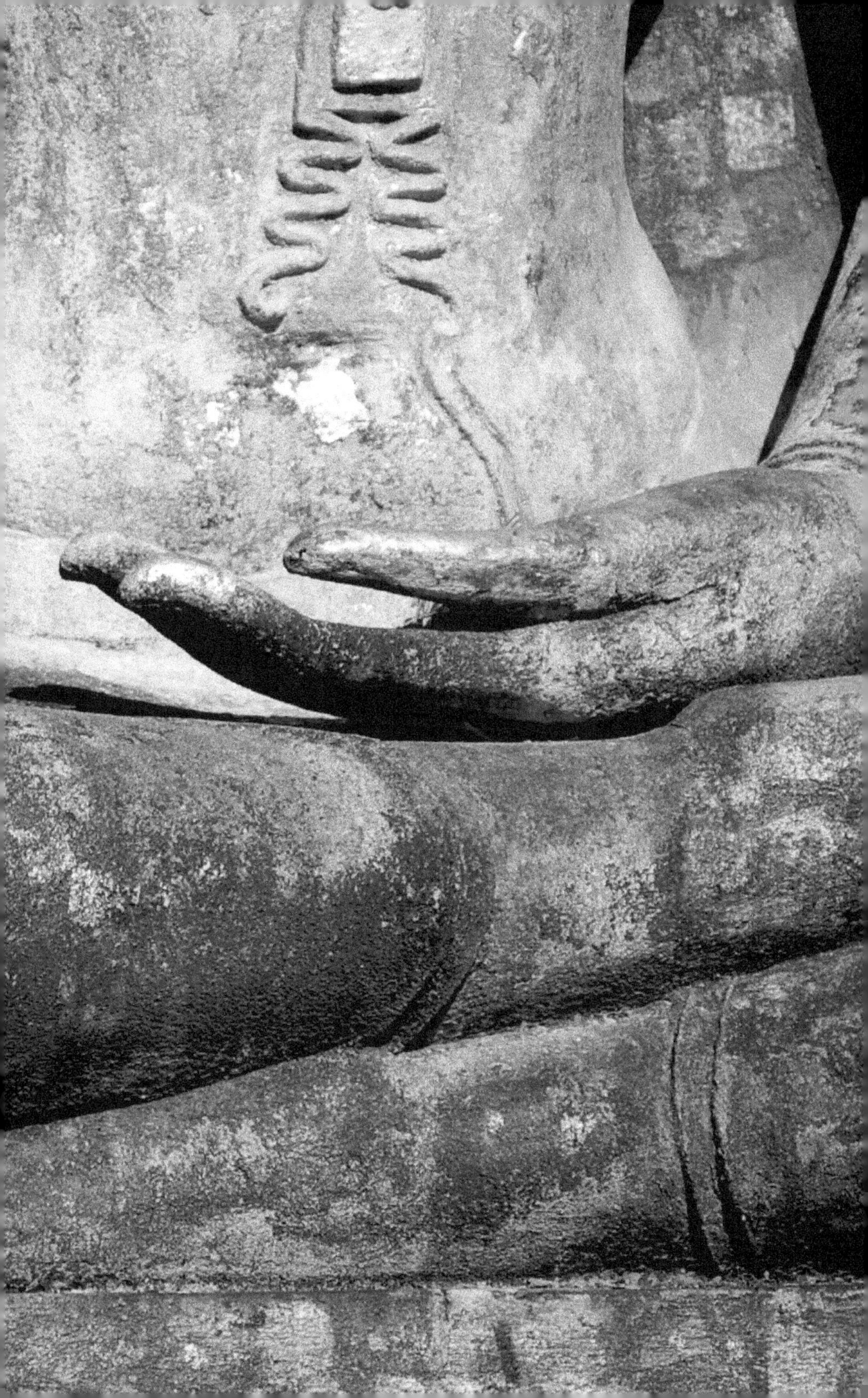

color red, which indicates fire and heat. The yantra is a red triangle. Agni is often called the "devouring force" and stands for instability. The power of fire is destructive but can be seen as a catalyst for change, development, and evolution. In our physical body, tattwa agni regulates our digestive fire, appetite, thirst, and sleep. It has its place between the heart and the navel. Its psychic centers are the Manipura chakra. The spiritual experience of the element is swar loka and manomaya kosha, our mental / thought body.

APAS TATTWA – the element of water.

Apas can be described as a large amount of intensively active matter that has emerged from agni tattwa. It is a matter that is not yet coherent, as the molecules and atoms are in great chaos. The universe is said to take the form of tattwa apas before it appears. Yantra, for the element, is a horizontal crescent surrounded by water. Our body can see apas through blood, mucus, bile, and lymph fluid as it controls our body fluids. The element affects our thoughts related to ourselves and worldly things. The apas has its seat between the navel and the knees. Mentally, it relates to our subconscious and conscious mind. Its psychic centers are the Swadhisthana chakra. The spiritual experience of tattwa apas is bhuvar loka and pranamaya kosha, our energy body.

PRITHVI TATTWA – the element of earth.

The last tattwa is prithvi, or bhumi, "to be". In prithvi, the motion of the particles has stopped almost completely. Energy has become matter in solid, liquid, or gas form. This element bears the yellow color, and the yantra is a yellow square. It has the qualities of firmness, weight, and cohesion. Our physical body can see this through bones and other organs. Since prithvi has emerged from all the other elements, it has all the qualities, but smell is the dominant quality. The component creates stability physically, mentally, and in our environment and stands for the material. It has its physical place between our toes and knees. Mentally, it relates to the conscious and subconscious mind. Its psychic center is the Mooladhara chakra. The spiritual experience of prithvi tattwa is bhu loka and annamaya kosha, our physical body.

TATTWAS AND KOSHAS

The elements build up layers that are called koshas in yoga. Man is said to have five layers, all of which vibrate differently and relate to different levels of consciousness. The first and coarsest layer is called annamaya kosha; our body is made of food. Pranamaya kosha is the layer of prana, manomaya kosha is the layer of thoughts, vijnamaya kosha is the layer of intuition, and the last layer is the layer of body bliss, anandamaya kosha.

These subtle layers of man can only be affected with the help of yoga, tantra, and other spiritual exercises. In tattwa shuddhi, annamaya kosha and pranamaya kosha are af-

fected by controlling respiration and increasing the flow of prana. Manomaya kosha is affected by concentration. Vijnamaya kosha is aroused by concentration on tattwa yantras. There is no direct exercise to influence anandamaya kosha. Working with the other four layers of bodies is necessary to experience anandamaya kosha.

Experiences of color, light, and smell during tattwa shuddhi are experiences of our subtle bodies.

Koshas are also linked to seven planes of consciousness. These are called lokas. Each loka relates to a plane of existence through which consciousness develops. The elements influence each loka, and through tattwa shuddhi, we also influence these.

TATTWAS AND BREATHING

Elements such as chitta Shakti, prana Shakti and atma Shakti are manifested in our physical body. These act in the body and mind through our energy channels, nadis or breathing (swara). Swara and nadi mean flow. Nadi is the flow of Shakti in our subtle body while swara shastra is the flow of our breathing in nadis. Swara shastra is thus the science behind the flow of breathing and nadis. The three Shakti that flow in our breath are channeled through three main nadis in the body (ida, pingala and sushumna). It is said that we have about seventy-two thousand nadis in the body. Ida, pingala, and sushumna are responsible for the psychosomatic and spiritual parts of the body, mind, and consciousness. Chitta Shakti, the power of ida nadi, is the vital and mental energy that controls all our functions regarding thoughts, mind, and chitta. All mental activity is the result of the flow of ida. This flow is connected to our left nostril and affects the right side of the brain. It is also called chandra swara and relates to the negative aspect of the energy in the body.

Prana Shakti flows through the pingala nadi. It is the vital life energy and relates to the positive aspect of it. Prana Shakti controls all physical activity. The flow of pingala nadi is connected to our right nostril and affects the left side of the cerebral hemisphere. It is also called surya swara. Atma Shakti is channeled through sushumna nadi—Pranan's central passage for spiritual consciousness. Sushumna is neutral energy active when breathing flows through both nostrils simultaneously. This condition affects the activity of the dormant parts of the brain. In our physical body, these three nadis relate to the parasympathetic (ida), sympathetic (pingala) and autonomic (sushumna) nervous systems. In most people, sushumna is closed for most of their lives, meaning ida and pingala control them. Through yogic and tantric exercises, one can open up sushumna nadi.

These three aspects of energy manifest in our breathing cycles. The flow lasts about an hour in each nostril. When the flow changes, the sushumna is open for a few seconds. In our flow of swara, the elements are included. Each element has a specific pranic frequency and affects various bodily functions. Tattwas cause the swara to flow in different directions and affect ida, pingala and sushumna. Ida and pingala nadi channel shakti to the chakras in the body and affect their vibration. The elements also affect the chakras in the body through breathing. Each chakra is dominated by one element – Mooladhara by the earth element, Swadhisthana by the water element, Manipura by the fire element, Anahata by the air element, and Vishuddhi by the air element. Just as breathing affects our mental, physical, and spiritual existence, so do the elements, through their different character, affect our state of mind, body, and consciousness.

Through various tantric and yogic techniques, it is possible to practice the feeling for which tattwa is active in the swara for the moment. A tattwa yogi can assess his physical, mental, emotional and spiritual condition in this way. Examples of exercises that practice the ability are trataka on tattwa yantras and sensations of the elements (color and shape) during the performance of naumukhi mudra, yoni mudra or shanmukhi mudra. The last-mentioned exercises practice our knowledge and experience of the elements as they work. You close the gates for external perception and simultaneously open up to the inner experience of color, sound, smell, and form.

MANTRA, YANTRA & MANDALA

The theory and philosophy behind tantra are closely intertwined with mantra, yantra, and mandala. Tantra is a philosophical and practical science whose sublime theories become effective through mantra, yantra, and mandala. The unique thing about tantra is that there is always an explanation and valuable exercise for each philosophy or theory. Mantra, yantra and mandala are used in all tantric exercises, also within tattwa shuddhi.

MANDALA

The word mandala means circle, and in Hindu and Buddhist rituals, it refers to a figure drawn on the ground or painted on a table that symbolizes the cosmic and celestial regions. A mandala is a meditation figure constructed of circles and shapes. Correctly depicted and properly inaugurated, it becomes a concentration of occult energy, which attracts hidden forces and emits rays like a talisman. Within the boundaries of the mandala circle, other geometric figures are drawn: smaller squares, triangles, and circles that divide it all into sacred zones.

To create a mandala, one must be able to see into oneself. Not by thinking – but by vision, as clearly and distinctly as with open eyes. The more precise the inner vision, the more influential the created mandala. The principle behind a mandala is that it exists in the form of a circle. The circle stands for the basic shape behind everything. Anything can shape a mandala, a tree, a house, a car, an animal, or a human being. Even the body is a mandala. To create a mandala that carries strength and power, one must be able to create an exact copy of the inner vision. A mandala is the essence of an object experienced by someone who has refined the inner eye, an inner cosmic image of which everyone can partake. The level of consciousness lays the foundation for what the mandala will look like. All forms of art, sculpture, and architecture are from the beginning mandala's given form.

In tantra, mandalas are also depicted as illustrated images of divine forces. A human form of the sacred makes it easier for the rough mind of man to understand and experience the power within when the ability to visualize is weak. The symbolism and structure behind the images of deities are intended to awaken the equivalent in the individual's consciousness. By concentrating on mandalas, deeply rooted samskaras are awakened within.

Perhaps the most talked about mandala created in tantra is maithuna kriya. Maithuna kriya forms a mandala that has corresponding yantras and mantras. The erotic sculptures of the Khajuraho Temple in Orissa are based on the tantric belief that maithuna is intended to awaken man's divine forces. The man represents Shiva, the physical energy, and the woman, Shakti, the mental energy. Mandalas are created as a force field or energy circle through their exoteric and esoteric union. Linga and yoni mandala are also symbols of this higher union. Man and woman physically unite to re-experience the unity from which they were created. This union is an inner experience in the same way as the spiritual experience.

YANTRA

A yantra is an abstract mathematical image of an inner vision. Behind each rough shape is a subtle shape, which the yantra represents. Everything in nature can be experienced in its original form (yantra). It carries an inherent energy just like everything else in creation. By visualizing and concentrating on the yantra, one can awaken the corresponding energy in oneself. The yantra comprises the primary and original shapes: a bindu / dot, a circle, a square, and a triangle. Bindu is the point from which everything has been created and to which everything will return; it is the process of creation and dissolution. It also represents the union between Shiva and Shakti. Bindu is also found in our body, on the top of the back of the head, and is called Bindu visarga. During meditation, one uses the outer Bindu as a yantra to experience the contraction of time and space in bindu in the physical body. The triangle stands for the first shape that comes out of creation and is also known as the moola tricona (spelling should be trikona in English). Upside down, it stands for Prakriti (creation), and with the tip facing upwards, it stands for Purusha (consciousness). The circle represents the cycle of timelessness where neither the beginning nor the end exists, only eternity. It symbolizes the process of birth, life, and death. The square is the base on which the yantra rests and represents the physical, earthly world that must be refined.

Yantras create a path from the outer to our inner. They are essential for our continued spiritual evolution: they strengthen our creative and intuitive sides and spiritual experiences. In tattwa shuddhi, one uses yantra created from the four primary forms.

MANTRA

In the same way that every thought has an equivalent in the form of an image, every image also has an equivalent in sound, nada, or vibration. These sounds are called mantras. Mantra means" contemplating what leads to liberation." Nada is one of the first manifestations of creation, the form. In Indian philosophy, it is believed that the first sound of creation was the sound of "Om," which is the cosmic mantra. Mandukyo Upanishad describes how the mantra affects and expands different levels of consciousness. "Om" is made up of three syllables, "A", "U", and "M", which all vibrate at different frequencies, which affect the consciousness in different ways. When you repeat "Om," you raise awareness to the same frequency as the mantra. It applies to all mantras.

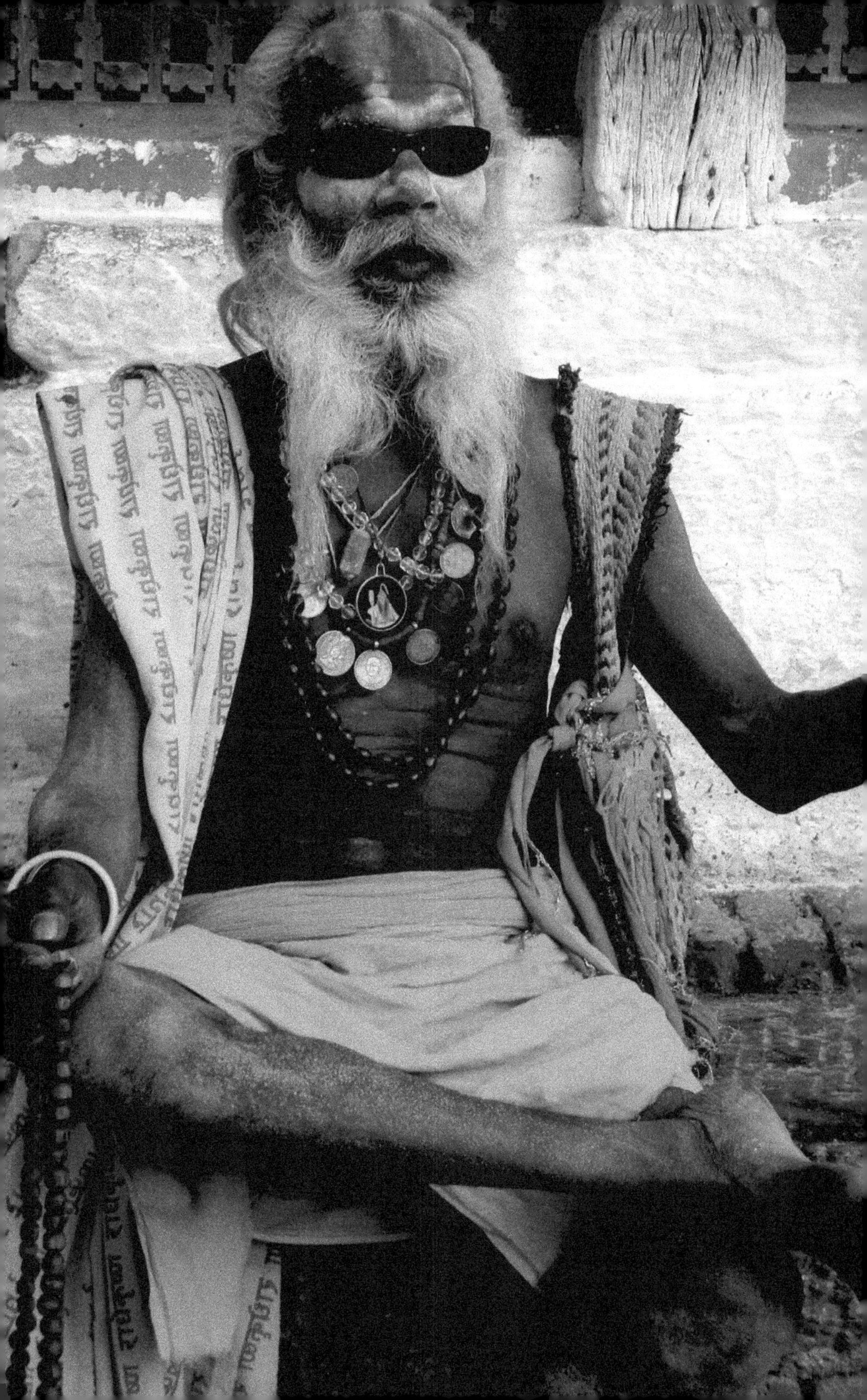

Nada consists of four frequencies: para (cosmic), pashyanti (temporary), madhyama (subtle) and vaikhari (rough) and correspond to the four frequency levels that "Om" carries: consciously, unconsciously, subconsciously and turya. The entire Sanskrit alphabet consists of mantras. In Sanskrit, the letters are not called letters but akshara, which means imperishable. Each akshara can be used as a mantra. Therefore, it is said that only by reading Vedas can one achieve liberation.

The most potent form of the mantra is the bija mantra. Bija means seed and is the sound from which all other mantras are derived. The Bija mantra is a powerful, concentrated energy attributed to different levels of consciousness. In tattwa shuddhi, bija mantras related to the five elements are used. Even in tantra, it is known that each physical body part has a mantra to which it corresponds. These mantras are used in nyasa to transform the physical body into a container for more extraordinary powers, which is aroused by tattwa shuddhi and other esoteric techniques.

Breathing has its mantra created by inhaling (So) and exhaling (Ham) and is known as the ajapa japa mantra. In the Upanishads, it is said that this mantra is powerful enough in itself to awaken Kundalini Shakti and expand consciousness. In the introduction to tattwa shuddhi, the mantra So Ham creates a sense of belonging to the universal consciousness.

By repeating the mantra, you raise the consciousness, and by concentrating on a yantra, you focus the consciousness to a point. At a level of consciousness, the inner experience manifests as a thought or emotion; at a higher level, it becomes an inner vision or mandala. It becomes a yantra later manifested as sound, nada, or mantra when you go deeper. When the mind functions under lower and coarser energy frequencies, it becomes static, sluggish, slow, and tamasic. When you make the energy more subtle through mantra, yantra, and mandala, the state of mind changes from tamasic to becoming rajasic and finally sattvic.

Mantras, yantras, and mandalas used in tattwa shuddhi have nothing to do with religion, occultism, or mysticism. They should be regarded as highly charged forces who intend to create the same frequency in man that the mantra, yantra, or mandala carries to raise consciousness.

VISUALIZATION AND FANTASY

To create, one must first and foremost be able to visualize and fantasize. Imagination is a mental ability that can be used in all ways. When you make an inner world of visions and symbols, the power of the mind becomes more robust. In tantra, visualization and imagination link the objective and subjective worlds. Tantric visualizations serve as a guide for the practitioner, a medium to concentrate on. In tattwa shuddhi, you want to make the practitioner experience their inner self by creating colors, sounds and images, and visu-alization of these in concrete form. The pictures are both grotesque and pleasant. The practitioner has clear guidelines to follow to help him reach deeper. In the beginning, you experience the images as thoughts, which, over time, develop into clear, inner images.

THE PERFORMANCE OF PAPA PURUSHA
– the sinful man.

The meditation exercises in tattwa shuddhi consist of many unusual fantasies. The most bizarre of these is Papa Pur-usha. Papa Purusha symbolizes the cause of suffering, conflict, disharmony and imbalance caused by ego, jealousy, pride, etc. During the exercise, you imagine how Papa Pur-usha is transformed and takes shape, meaning you change yourself. Papa Purusha's transformation refers to the inner transformation. The transformation and conflict between the negative and positive forces (ida and pingala) constantly stri-ve to unite and transform into the third neutral force. This conflict acts as a catalyst for our evolution and causes us to continue to seek balance in life. In our search for balance, we turn to the spiritual paths, which guide our evolution further and further forward. We would remain complacent and lazy without the conflict between the opposites of energies. Tantra emphasizes the importance of experiencing conflict to create harmony.

The performance of papa purusha is covered on the stage during the exercise when you have become the experience. You witness every action and thought. Each reaction is assessed objectively. Only then, when one can look at oneself objectively, can one see the sides of one's personality that the ego has previously hidden, ages you would rather not see or know about. Here, too, tantra emphasizes the importance of daring to see oneself as one is, not as one wants to be. Only then do you have the opportunity to change yourself.

BHASMA

Tattwa shuddhi is a symbolic act where one lubricates the body with ash (bhasma) to cleanse the body physically and subtly. The great yogi Shiva, the father of tantra, is often depicted sitting naked and anointed in ashes. Lubricating oneself with bhasma favors the experience and discovery of one's own Shiva nature.

Bhasma means "dissolution" or "decomposition" and refers to the decomposition of matter using fire or water. The "bhasmatic" form of matter is produced, which is considered a purer and finer form than the original and all impurities disappear. All matter must finally undergo this process to transform into the fine essential form. It also applies to us humans. To cleanse means the elimination of slag and impurities. The application of bhasma symbolizes our inner consciousness's journey from rough matter to pure consciousness.

Bhasma is also used in Ayurveda as a medical treatment method. Bhasma can be made of gold, silver, copper, or other metals. In tattwa shuddhi, cow dung is used. Cow dung is used in India daily as it is considered antibacterial, antiviral, and generally beneficial to the skin. The reason why you use cow dung in tattwa shuddhi and no other substance is essential. By dissolving the cow dung with the help of agni (fire) one reduces it to its bhasmatic form which symbolizes the dissolution of our senses which we try to do in tattwa shuddhi. Through pratyahara, we loosen up the experience of the objective world and our surroundings. Through dharana, we concentrate the knowledge of what is left to experience, and through dhyana, we broaden this experience to its original cosmic essence, the Shiva consciousness.

In tattwa shuddhi, bhasma is applied to the forehead at the same time as the mantra is pronounced towards the end of the exercise—most people who have done this experience feeling deeply cleansed. Rishis and yogis have used bhasma throughout the ages, and its beneficial effect has led to the technology being used even today.

THE EFFECT OF TATTWA SHUDDHI SADHANA

The effects of tattwa shuddhi are faster and more powerful when compared to other sadhana, as it is a tantric upasana that one dedicates to Shakti, the energy principle behind everything. The effects manifest themselves both materially and as mental forces (siddhis). However, it is essential to remember to perform tattwa shuddhi correctly so as not to create imbalances and obstacles that interfere with the continued spiritual development. It is important to learn the technique from a knowledgeable teacher or guru. Regularity is essential for the exercise, different from how often you practice. We want to train the mind, intellect, and consciousness in tantra. We want to be able to control it with our willpower. It teaches us that regular practice is essential.

PHYSICALLY

The combination of fasting and tattwa shuddhi contributes to changes throughout our physical body. When we cleanse the elements (tattwas) that our body is built of, our heart, liver, kidneys, pancreas and all other organs are affected. Tissues and cells are renewed and given new energy, contributing to a healthier body and mind. Bhasma has a cooling effect on the body and nervous system, which can be heated during intense meditation.

MENTALLY

By visualizing and concentrating on tattwa yantras, chanting mantras, and creating mandalas, we purify samskaras that can be manifested through dreams, visions, and thoughts in our conscious mind. Mental visions are a common effect of most yogic exercises, but within tattwa shuddhi these are usually stronger when one has developed a sharp inner cons-

ciousness. You can experience these as subtle sounds, smells, a feeling on the skin, or as taste and shape.

SIDDHIS

Yoga shastras clearly describe that siddhis can be achieved by concentrating on tattwas. By awakening tattwas, one develops higher abilities such as clairvoyance, telepathy, and intuition. The earth's elements help cure diseases and make the body light. Apas tattwa evens the flow of prana in the body and enables astral travel. Agni tattwa can turn base metals into precious metals. Vayu tattwa provides knowledge about the past, present, and future. Akasha tattwa develops mental projection and reveals metaphysical reality. Despite this, siddhis are not what we strive for in tattwa shuddhi; the purpose is higher spiritual experiences that involve the knowledge of the subtle forces that permeate the entire universe. You thus become more receptive to these forces. You naturally become more intuitive and experience bliss on all levels. In tantric texts, one can also read that the knowledge of the elements leads one to freedom from suffering. It is done by knowing that all matter is perishable and that the human body results from atoms, molecules, and energy particles. You stop attaching to things and matter when you know what they consist of – i.e., composite energy.

TATTWA SHUDDHI

PERFORMANCE

Before you start practicing tattwa shuddhi, you and your teacher / guru should take a sankalpa regarding how long and often you should practice. It is said that a sankalpa should be as short as one day. The person's willpower and mental ability should be considered when determining the period. A sankalpa must always be completed. You can start practicing at any time during the year, but it is said that July-August (Shravan) or October (Ashwin, the month of devi worship) gives the best results.

It would help if you looked after your diet during exercise. Heavy food makes the body sluggish and slow, is difficult for the body to digest, and can make it harder to be receptive to higher energies. Salt, solid spices, and beverages should be avoided as they increase digestion and can cause too much acid to form. Light foods like dairy products, fruits, and cooked vegetables are preferred. If you have decided to do tattwa shuddhi daily, or for some other reason can not keep a light diet, you should adjust the diet to what is best suited. The special requirements regarding fasting and diet do not need to be followed if one does not have a strict sadhana and only practices tattwa shuddhi once a day.

According to tradition, tattwa shuddhi should be practiced three times a day. During Brahma muhurta (before sunrise), afternoon, and sandhya (dusk). Before the exercise, wash yourself. You should practice in a quiet, calm place with few impressions and sit facing north or east. Before the exercise, light a candle and read out your sankalpa. During the last day, practice mouna, and after the previously completed exercise, sit and meditate on the formless reality.

Step 1: Preparation.

Practice trataka or pranayama for ten to fifteen minutes before the exercise to calm the mind and go deeper into yourself (pratyahara).

Sit in a comfortable meditation position, close your eyes, and practice kaya sthairyam.

Visualize the form of your guru or spiritual guide and feel reverence for them.

Take your attention to the Mooladhara chakra and imagine how the Kundalini Shakti rises upwards with the sushumna nadi to the Sahasrara chakra on top of the head. Meditate on the mantra So Ham, synchronize with breathing: So on inhalation, from Mooladhara to Sahasrara, and Ham on exhalation from Sahasrara to Mooladhara. Experience the movement of the mantra and the breathing as if it were the movement of your inner consciousness.

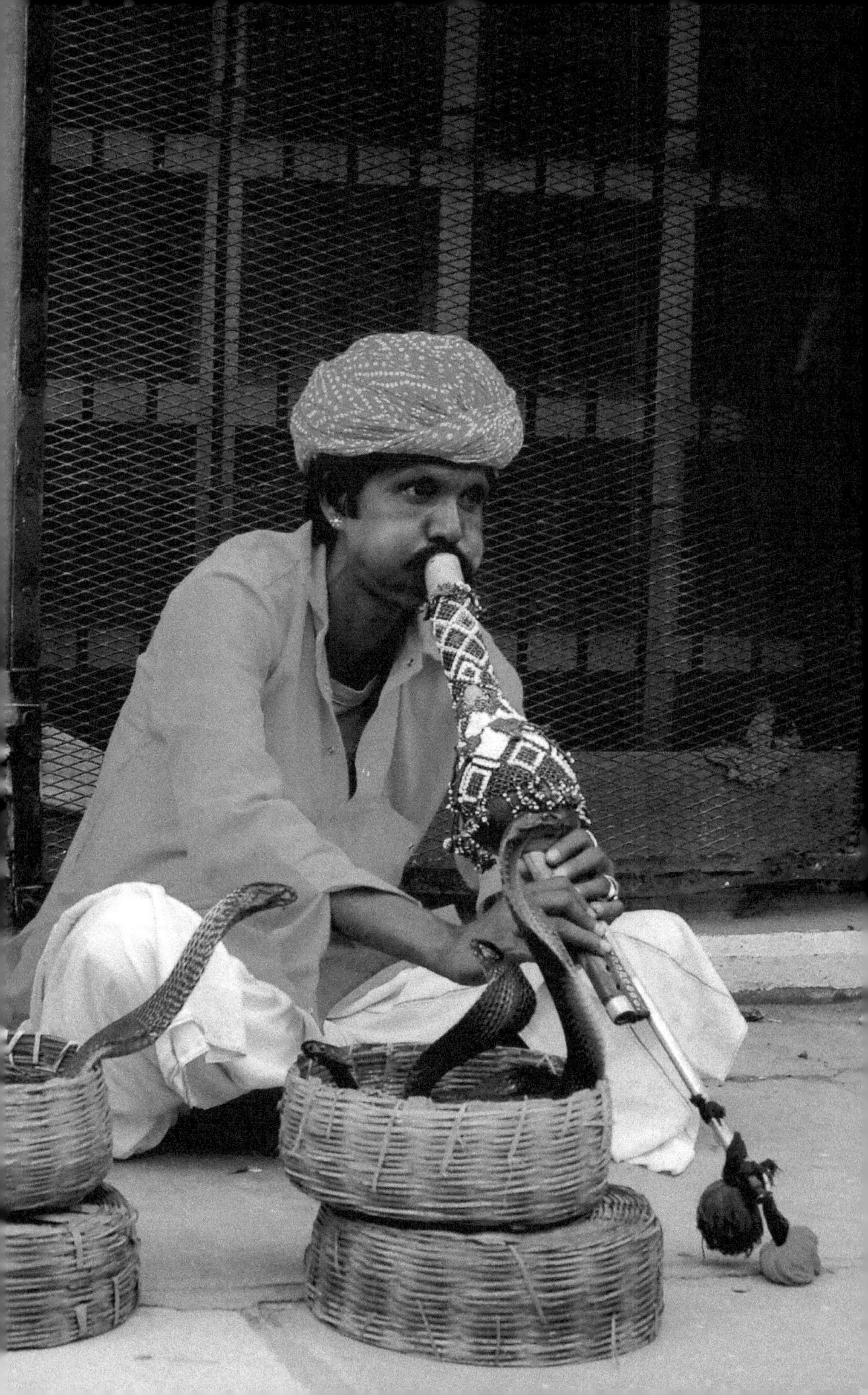

Step 2: The creation of tattwa yantras.

Take consciousness to the area between the toes and knees. Visualize the shape of a yellow square, the yantra for prithvi tattwa, the earth's element. Experience its golden yellow color and weight. At the same time, repeat the bija mantra, Lam.

Move your attention to the area between the knees and the navel. Visualize a horizontal crescent moon with two white lotus flowers at each end. A circle of water surrounds the crescent. It is the yantra of the apas tattwa, the element of water. Repeat with the mantra Vam.

Move the attention further to the area between the navel and the heart. Visualize a red upside-down triangle burning, the yantra for agni tattwa, the element of fire. Simultaneously repeat the mantra Ram.

Now, focus on the area between the heart and the eyebrow center. Visualize a blue hexagon, which is yantra for the vayu tattwa. Repeat with the mantra Yam.

Move your attention to the area between the eyebrow's center and the head's top. Imagine a circle, the yantra of akasha tattwa, the element of space / ether. In the circle is shoonya (the emptiness), black or filled with multicolored dots. Repeat the mantra, Ham.

Step 3: Resolution of the elements.

Take consciousness back to prithvi yantra. Experience how its form becomes fluid and turns into apas, apas into agni, agni into vayu, and vayu into akasha.

Now imagine how the aksha is transformed into its origin, the ahamkara, the ego.

The ego is then transformed into the mahat tattwa, the great principle. Mahat tattwa dissolves and becomes Prakriti, Prakriti to Purusha (the highest self).

Consider yourself the highest principle, pure and complete.

Step 4: Transformation of the lower nature.

Pay attention to the left side of the abdomen / stomach. Visualize there a tiny man as big as your thumb. He is called Papa Purusha. His skin was black as soot, and he had glowing eyes and a big belly. He holds an ax in one hand and a shield in the other. He is grotesque in form. You will now transform this man with the help of breathing and mantras.

Hold the right nostril with your right thumb and inhale through the left nostril. At the same time, repeat the mantra Yam four times. Visualize how his face and body transform.

Hold both nostrils. Hold your breath and, at the same time, repeat the mantra Ram four times. See how the little man is burned to ashes.

Exhale the ashes through your right nostril while repeating the mantra Vam four times. See how the ashes are rolled into a ball mixed with the moon's nectar in the apas yantra.

Now repeat the mantra, Lam. Imagine how the ball on the left side of your stomach transforms into a golden egg.

Repeat the mantra Ham and simultaneously visualize how the golden egg grows in size and fills your whole body. It feels like you are born again.

Step 5: Re-formation of the elements.

Reshape the elements in reverse order. You again become the highest principle from the golden egg, Prakriti, mahat tattwa, ahamkara.

From ahamkara you see how akasha yantra is created, from akasha is created vayu, from vayu is created agni, from agni is created apas, from apas is created prithvi.

Locate the area for each tattwa yantra and repeat the mantra for each tattwa as before.

Step 6: Kundalini back to Mooladhara.

When you have recreated all the elements, repeat the mantra So Ham along with the sushumna synchronized with the breathing. Move the attention from Mooladhara to Sahasrara and from Sahasrara to Mooladhara.

Experience how you, with the separation of jivatma (your soul), separate from paramatma (the cosmic soul). Place jivatma at the heart of its location.

Visualize the Kundalini Shakti that you directed to the Sahasrara and experience how it returns down to the Mooladhara through the sushumna while piercing each chakra on the way down.

Step 7: The shape of the shakti.

Bring your attention to chidakasha. See a giant deep sea in front of you with a large red lotus flower on the water. On the lotus flower, see the shape of prana Shakti.

Her body is the same color as a sunrise and decorated with ornaments. She has three eyes and six arms. In her first hand, she holds a trident; in the second, a bow made of sugar cane; in the third, a snare; in the fourth, a spur; in the fifth, five arrows; and the sixth, a skull with blood dripping from it.

Look at her beautiful shape and say, "May she give us happiness."

Step 8: Application of bhasma.

Become aware of yourself sitting on the floor. Become body conscious. Inhale slowly and deeply. Open your eyes.

Take some bhasma on the middle and ring fingers and slowly pull the fingers on the forehead from left to right while pronouncing the mantra "Om Hraum Namah Shivaya" or "Om Ham Sa" (Sannyasins).

Take bhasma on your thumb, draw a line above the other two lines from right to left, and pronounce the same mantra again.

Did you like the book? Feel free to follow me on my social media, share and like, tell your friends about the books, and feel free to write an honest review; one or two lines don't matter. All support is precious. Thanks!

On my Facebook page and Instagram, I post exciting news and tips on temporary offers and benefits you can take advantage of. I often also post my yoga routine and other things related to nutrition and health that may be interesting to take part in. So feel free to join them so you don't miss anything interesting:

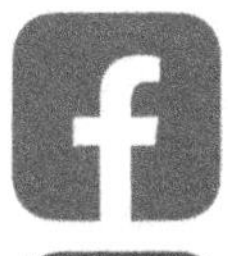 *facebook.com/bhagwanoneofakindbooks*

 *instagram.com/bhagwanoneofakindbooks/*

MY BOOKS AND BOOK SERIES

I have two book series that have different audiences. Great Yoga Books – is a series with the most comprehensive fact books on yoga for those who want to explore the subject in depth. Here, you will also find classic yoga books that are rarely translated, such as Patanjali's Yoga Sutras and Hatha Yoga Pradipika. My second series, Yoga Beyond the Poses: The Ultimate Beginner's Guide to Yoga, covers one yoga topic at a time and is extra easy to read with larger text. For those who find it challenging to read extensive books and want a good and broad overview of the subject quickly. Both series are also available as audiobooks.

★★★★★

TEACHING YOGA
&
MEDITATION
BEYOND
THE POSES

BESTSELLING AUTHOR

Shreyananda
Natha

Teaching Yoga and Meditation Beyond the Poses – A unique and practical workbook!

Teaching Yoga and Meditation Beyond the Poses – A unique and practical workbook for aspiring yoga teachers who want to teach yoga and meditation beyond the poses.

Teaching Yoga and Meditation Beyond the Poses is a unique and essential resource for new and experienced teachers and a guide for all yoga students interested in refining their skills and knowledge. Teaching Yoga and Meditation is also ideal as a core textbook in yoga teacher training programs.

The book covers fundamental yoga philosophy and history topics, including a historical presentation of classical yoga literature: Yoga Sutras of Patanjali, Bhagavad Gita, etc. Each of the seven major styles of yoga is described, from Hatha yoga, Raja yoga, Tantra yoga, Bhakti yoga, and Kundalini yoga, to knowledge about the chakras, Ayurveda and magic mantras and yantras. The book provides extensive support and tools for teaching integrated and classical yoga (asanas), breathing techniques (pranayama), deep relaxation (Yoga Nidra), and meditation (Ajapa Japa). The book is divided into eight modules with associated knowledge tests and complete yoga and meditation classes.

https://rb.gy/9s6edj

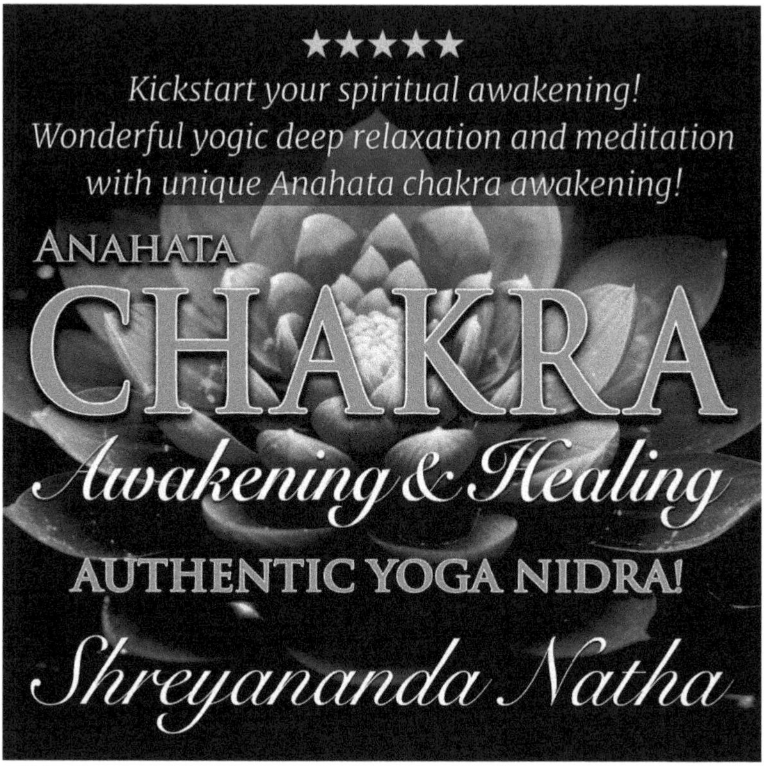

★★★★★

Kickstart your spiritual awakening!
Wonderful yogic deep relaxation and meditation
with unique Anahata chakra awakening!

ANAHATA
CHAKRA
Awakening & Healing
AUTHENTIC YOGA NIDRA!
Shreyananda Natha

Download the **AUDIOBOOK** here!
SCAN QR-CODE or go to:
https://bit.ly/3Hm7EQc

9 789198 839258